DISCARD

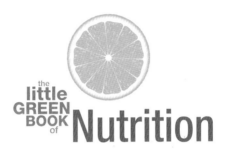

the
little
GREEN
BOOK
of **Nutrition**

For Nick – thanks for your love and support.

Text and design copyright © 2008
Carlton Books Limited

This edition published by
Carlton Books Limited 2008
20 Mortimer Street
London W1T 3JW

ISBN 978-1-84732-225-8

Printed and bound in Singapore

Senior Executive Editor: Lisa Dyer
Senior Art Editor: Gulen Shevki-Taylor
Designer: Emma Wicks
Copy Editor: Nicky Gyopari
Production: Kate Pimm

Your **Carbon Footprint** is the amount of carbon dioxide emitted
due to your daily activities – from washing a load of laundry to
buying air-freighted vegetables. See www.carbonfootprint.com
for ways to reduce your impact on the environment.

DIANE MILLIS

the
little
GREEN
BOOK
of
Nutrition

250 TIPS FOR AN ECO LIFESTYLE

CARLTON
BOOKS

Global food and agricultural systems account for up to 30% of all human-induced global warming – and food is responsible for 31% of the average European household's impact on climate change, so the foods you choose matter for the environment.

1 DO YOUR HOMEWORK

If you really want to make sure your food and drink choices are positive for the environment as well as for your health, then do your research and beware those that over-simplify. Buying local, for example, isn't always the greenest choice – while there are high carbon emissions associated with flying green beans in from Kenya, you might find that overall more carbon emissions come from growing green beans nearer to home due to an intensive system of agriculture used that relies on machinery, fertilizers, heating, irrigation systems and so on.

2 LABEL QUICK-FIX

Carbon footprint labels are starting to be used on products, but assessment is complex … Do you count how long the product sits in the store refrigerator? Do you include non-carbon, but powerful, global warming emissions such as methane from cattle? Buying less of most items is still the best thing you can do for your carbon footprint.

3 FARMING MATTERS

Farmers can now use an online tool (www.cla.org.uk) to measure their farms' greenhouse gas emissions – before you buy, ask if they are doing so.

4 SAVVY LOCAL SOURCING

Buying local means you can find out more about the way in which your food is produced – direct from the grower – and pick the producer who is doing the most to reduce their emissions. Look online for local producer guides, such as www.bigbarn.co.uk.

5 WASTE NOT, WANT NOT

The more food you buy directly from a producer the better in terms of waste. It is estimated that 40% of food never makes it from harvest to our plates as it's lost somewhere in the distribution network thanks to processing, storage and transportation.

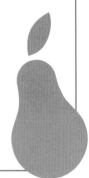

6 PUT IT ON THE LIST

As a green tool it's pretty basic and it has been around for years, but a shopping list really will help keep food waste down and your healthy eating plans on track. If you are one of the third of all shoppers who doesn't check what food you need before heading to the shops or take a list with you, then get writing.

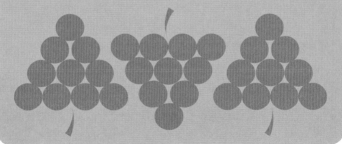

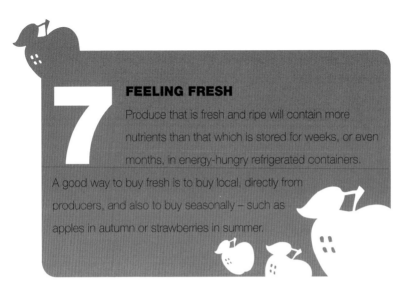

7 FEELING FRESH

Produce that is fresh and ripe will contain more nutrients than that which is stored for weeks, or even months, in energy-hungry refrigerated containers. A good way to buy fresh is to buy local, directly from producers, and also to buy seasonally – such as apples in autumn or strawberries in summer.

8 VIRTUALLY LOCAL

For the average time-pressed person, the idea of visiting several different stores each week in order to get all you need locally just isn't realistic but there are other ways to shop locally. Local Food Shop (www.localfoodshop.co.uk) is an online service that lets British consumers search by postcode for suppliers in their region, and producers based close to each other are encouraged to team up and combine deliveries. In the US, visit www.localharvest.org to find farmers' markets, family farms and other sources of sustainably grown food in your area.

9 CREATE A POCKET MARKET

In the US, a regional food cooperative has introduced the idea of 'pocket markets'. Smaller than farmers' markets – sometimes just two or three stalls – they sell produce from local farmers, local urban growers and community gardeners. Communities provide the location and volunteers run the stalls. See www.foodroots.ca/pmtoolkit_index.htm for ideas on getting one going in your area.

10 OPT FOR ORGANIC

Studies show that, on average, organic food contains more vitamins and minerals than non-organic, and organic plants can contain between 10 and 15% more phenolics (compounds that are thought to help prevent diseases). In the case of organic fruit and vegetables, this is likely to be because plants grow in a naturally nutrient-rich soil. Another recent study found that organic fruit and vegetables contain higher levels of beneficial minerals such as iron and zinc.

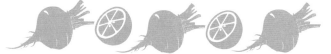

11 LESS EMISSIONS

Eating organic could also result in lower CO_2 emissions. A recent UK Government study found that organic production led to a 26% reduction in carbon emissions; other studies have shown that CO_2 emissions from organic farming are 40–60% lower per hectare than conventional systems, mainly because organic farmers do not use synthetic nitrogen fertilizers.

12 THINK ABOUT WATER

You need to take water into account when looking into the environmental impact of your food. According to the Food Ethics Council (www.foodethicscouncil.org), the world uses 200 million litres (53 million gallons) of water a second to grow its food but, by 2025, an estimated 1.8 billion people will be living without enough water to survive. In fact, agriculture uses 70% of the world's water, rising to 90% in many developing countries, and wastes 60% of the water it uses each year. Read the World Wildlife Fund's report on 'Thirsty Crops' at www.wwf.org.uk.

13 IGNORE THE DEALS

While food prices continue to rise, the temptation to 'buy one get one free' is going to be even greater but these deals are often a big factor in the amount of food that is wasted, especially when they are applied to perishable foods. Don't be drawn into buying more than you need unless you know that you are going to be able to freeze whatever's left.

14 BUY FAIRTRADE

Fairly traded products guarantee that disadvantaged producers in the developing world are getting a better deal by receiving a minimum price that covers the cost of sustainable production as well as an extra premium that's invested in social or economic development projects. Tea, coffee, bananas and chocolate are good examples of fairly traded products. Look out for certification by Fairtrade Labelling Organizations International (FLO).

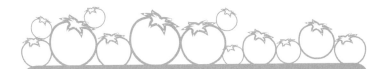

15 IS BIODYNAMIC BEST?

Biodynamic agriculture is a sustainable way in which to grow food since every biodynamic farm aims to become self-sufficient – in compost, manures and animal feeds. In 2002, a Swiss study showed that biodynamically tended soil has a higher biodiversity than either conventionally or organically farmed soil. For biodynamic produce look out for the Demeter symbol.

16 GO SLOW

Find out about 'slow food'. The Slow Food Movement began in Italy in the 1980s as an antidote to fast food and today the 'eco-gastronomy' movement has over 85,000 members in 132 countries. It seeks to retain the diverse heritage of regional food and drink and protect it from globalization, while also promoting biodiversity through its Slow Food Foundation for Biodiversity. See www.slowfood.com – and get involved.

17 A WORTHWHILE TRADE?

International trade can bring questionable benefits but it can also result in huge greenhouse gas emissions. For example, in 2006 the amount of beer the UK sold in Spain was almost the same as the amount Spain sold in the UK. Are we demanding choice for the sake of it? Make your food and drink choices local and sustainable.

18 SHIPPING ISN'T SHIP-SHAPE

Picking shipped produce over air-freighted is not the answer to our environmental woes. In 2008, it was discovered that greenhouse gas emissions from shipping are nearly three times higher than previously believed. Emissions from shipping account for 5% of total annual emmissions compared to the aviation industry's 2% a year.

19 DON'T BE FOOLED BY BIOFUEL

Did you know that biofuels are likely to do just as much, if not more, environmental harm than conventional fuels and are leading to food shortages for the poor? Huge areas of land are now being used to grow biofuels such as soya, palm and sugar cane. A recent US study found that growing biofuel on converted rainforests, peatlands, savannas or grasslands created up to 420 times more CO_2 than it saved.

20 ONLINE BENEFITS

Buy online and be more systematic about what and how much you buy. Use some of the better search options now available that let you source 'seasonal' or 'locally produced' food. Plus, many supermarkets are starting to make deliveries with electric vans. In the case of Tesco in the UK, one store's electric home-delivery fleet saves 100 tonnes of CO_2 per year.

21 GET LABEL-WISE

It's easy to be mystified by the plethora of labels on foods. There's the traffic light system for fat, sugar and salt content, the Guideline Daily Amounts labels, a wide variety of food assurance schemes – such as the RSPCA's 'Freedom Food', organic certification symbols and so on. Get help decoding labels – try *Which?*'s food shopping card (www.which.co.uk) and the Food Standards Agency guide to labelling terms (www.eatwell.gov.uk).

22 DON'T START THE CAR

The weekly food shop is something many of us do in the car – in fact, shopping accounts for 20% of car journeys in the UK, and 12% of the distance covered. But driving just 10.5 km (6.5 miles) to the supermarket emits more carbon than flying a pack of Kenyan green beans to the UK. Buying more local food should allow you to walk and/or cycle to the shops and this exercise will help your health, too.

23 IN THE BAG

About 13 billion plastic bags are given away at supermarket checkouts each year in Britain – but they take anything from 400–1,000 years to break down, while paper bags use four to six times as much energy to produce. For a green option, use a reusable fairtrade, organic cotton bag.

24 ROLL ALONG

Go one better than taking your own bags to the checkout – buy a shopping trolley (shopping bag on wheels) and let it take the strain on your walk to the supermarket. You will be much more likely to ditch the car if you know you're not going to be putting your back out hauling your food home again. And they aren't as old-fashioned as they used to be – check out www.rollser.co.uk or get a traditional willow basket on wheels at www.englishwillowbaskets.co.uk.

25

GO UNPACKAGED

Look out for stores that let you buy goods in bulk and use your own containers. In the UK, one store – Unpackaged – operates in London selling hundreds of loose products from herbs and spices to eggs and bread (http://beunpackaged.com).

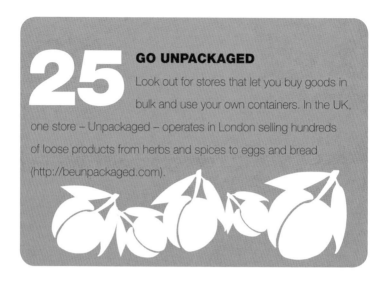

26

NEW IS NOT ALWAYS NICE

Each year the food and drink industry launches around 10,000 new products – most of which require huge amounts of the earth's resources to manufacture, package, distribute and dispose of. Don't become a slave to the industry's marketing departments – stick to the least processed and packaged foods, which have been providing good nutrition for years.

27 BEWARE ECO-HYPE

Nearly every company now claims it is becoming more climate-friendly but a lot of them aren't really making a concrete contribution when it comes to their overall impact on global warming. Supermarkets, for instance, might finally be doing something about giving away free plastic bags but they still use huge of amounts of energy in their stores and distribution network, and their businesses are based on selling lots of processed and imported food.

28 PICK THE BEST

If you must shop in a multiple, and 72% of UK grocery sales takes place in supermarkets, then at least ensure you are supporting the best green performer. Find out how UK supermarkets are doing against a list of green indicators in the National Consumer Council report 'Green grocers: how supermarkets can help make greener shopping easier' which it updates every few years – www.ncc.org.uk.

29

JUST GREENWASH?

If you are in search of green, nutritious food you will find yourself in a world of marketing hype, also known as 'greenwash' (dubious claims to eco-friendliness). Surveys in the UK and USA show that 9 out of 10 of us are sceptical about green or climate change information from companies and governments. Check what's behind the claims online – see the Greenwash Guide (www.futerra.co.uk/services/greenwash-guide).

30

BUY ETHICAL

Make sure the food and drink you buy has been made with wellbeing in mind. Ask for a manufacturer's and retailer's ethical policy (ideally, they will be members of the Ethical Trading Initiative). For the UK, take a look at Ethical Consumer's online guide (www.ethiscore.org), which rates companies against environmental, animal welfare and human rights issues. For the US, visit www.coopamerica.org/programs/responsibleshopper.

31 SET UP A GROUP

If you know a group of like-minded people (or want to get to know some) then consider setting up a local food group. In the UK, the Soil Association has produced a toolkit to help people establish an organic buying group – see www.localfoodworks.org, while in the US, Ecotrust has released 'Building Local Food Networks: A Toolkit for Organizers' (www.ecotrust.org).

32 THE MACROBIOTIC METHOD

Eating according to macrobiotic principles (developed by a Japanese philosopher in the 1920s) will bring down your carbon footprint as well as potentially your weight. The macrobiotic diet consists of foods that tend to be lacking in the average British or North American diet, such as fibre-rich wholegrains, vegetables and beans, while being low in saturated fat, meat, dairy products and sugar. It also emphasizes locally sourced, organic food.

33

CREATE A COMPOST

A heap of rotting food scraps, newspaper and green waste from your garden might not sound like a nutrition tip but it is if you use the resulting compost on your vegetable garden or allotment. Around 30% of each household's waste could be composted, but much of it ends up in landfill where it produces the powerful greenhouse gas methane. Throw it all on a compost heap and in around six months' time you'll get your very own natural fertilizers, mulch and soil conditioner. There are loads of online tips for would-be composters out there including www.recyclenow.com or www.howtocompost.org.

34

BUY A DIGESTER

For your cooked food waste consider investing in a food digester, which doesn't produce compost – it just breaks the food down until there is minimal residue – or try a Green Johanna 'hot' composter, which does produce compost.

35 CHEMICAL SOUP

Being at the top of the food chain, we are particularly exposed to chemicals in food, and research has found that oily fish and fatty foods, such as meat and dairy products, contain higher levels of chemicals like organochlorine pesticides, PCBs and flame retardants. These can cause cancer and birth defects, and damage the nervous system, so reduce the chemical burden on your body by buying organic.

36 TOP TEN TO AVOID

The charity Pesticide Action Network UK has devised a list of foods that are likely to have the highest pesticide residues. They are: flour, potatoes, bread, apples, pears, grapes, strawberries, green beans, tomatoes and cucumber. Consider buying these foods only if they are organic. In the US, the Organic Center has also produced a guide ('Organic Essentials' at www.organic-center.org).

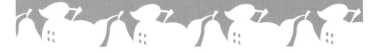

37 CONTAINER CONCERN

Avoid buying canned food and drinks in hard plastic polycarbonate bottles as they have been found to leach a chemical – Bisphenol A (BPA) – which can act like a female hormone and could be linked to breast cancer. In Canada, the use of BPA in plastic baby bottles has been banned, while recent US tests found that the lining in canned foods can leach more than double the amount of BPA than polycarbonate bottles.

38 USE WHAT YOU'VE GOT

We all waste a terrible amount of food – in the UK, for example, 6.7 million tonnes of food hits the bin each year, roughly a third of everything we buy. But not all of this waste is out of date or inedible. Organize your cooking so that you are eating food while it's fresh and use your imagination when it comes to using up the odds and ends in your fridge. You will also find ideas online – try www.lovefoodhatewaste.com.

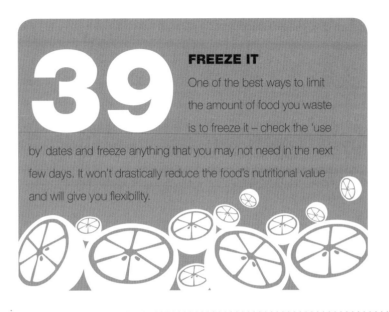

39 FREEZE IT

One of the best ways to limit the amount of food you waste is to freeze it – check the 'use by' dates and freeze anything that you may not need in the next few days. It won't drastically reduce the food's nutritional value and will give you flexibility.

40 PASS ON THE PROCESSING

Ready meals have crept onto many people's shopping lists. In the UK, 30% of adults eat ready-meals once a week, but they are rarely the best nutritional or eco-friendly option. Cooking and preservation processes ensure the nutritional content of most are low, while packaging and transporting them huge distances releases large amounts of carbon into the atmosphere, to say nothing of their contribution to our waste mountain.

41

WHEN PROCESSING IS GOOD

Occasionally processed food can improve the nutritional benefits of food – take tomatoes, for instance. They contain a powerful antioxidant – lycopene – but the body can access more of this nutrient if the tomato has been cooked. Indeed, there's five times more available lycopene in tomato sauce than in an equivalent amount of fresh tomatoes. But pick an organic ketchup or sauce and, if at all possible, one made locally.

42

SANDWICH SOLUTIONS

If you routinely buy pre-prepared sandwiches from a supermarket then it's time you thought about making your own. Apart from saving on the packaging waste and food miles (a recent study showed prepacked sandwiches sold in England often came from France), you will be able to liven up your taste buds by packing homemade sandwiches with nutritional goodies such as sprouts and avocado.

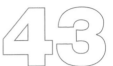

IT'S THE WAY IT'S MADE

A recent US study found that food production accounts for 83% of the 8.1 tonnes of greenhouse gases that an average US household generates each year by consuming food, while the transportation of food led to only 11% of total emissions. Different food groups varied widely in their emissions, with red meat, for example, producing 150% more greenhouse gases than chicken or fish. So it may well be better to cut your meat consumption rather than your food miles.

GENETIC DOUBTS

GM food is being heralded as a solution to food shortages and rising prices but environmental campaigners are still adamant that they pose a huge risk to wildlife. According to Friends of the Earth, two out of three GM crops grown in UK government-sponsored farm-scale trials were more damaging to farmland wildlife than their conventional equivalents. The group also says that most GM crops have resulted in increased pesticide use.

45 GENES IN YOUR FOOD

Routine trials for the unexpected health effects of GM food is not required before GMOs can be sold as food or grown in the open countryside, and at least four independent studies have found negative health effects. Newcastle University research found that genes from GM soya entered the gut bacteria of those eating it.

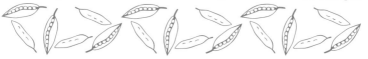

46 ORGANIC IS YOUR BEST BET

Ensuring you have a GM-free diet can be a challenge. In the US, GM foods and products are currently not labelled and roughly 70% of the foods in supermarkets have GM ingredients (see www.truefoodnow.org/shoppersguide). In the EU, products have to be labelled if they are from a GM source, but not if they have been produced with GM technology or come from animals fed on GM animal feed.

47 'E'S AREN'T GOOD

About 400 'E' number additives and several thousand un-named flavouring agents are used in our food. There is evidence that mixtures of artificial food colourings and a commonly used food preservative can increase hyperactive behaviour in susceptible children (see www.actiononadditives.com and www.foodcomm.org.uk). Buy fresh food only, and dry up the demand for these chemicals.

48 ADDITIVES TO LOOK OUT FOR

The US pressure group Center for Science in the Public Interest (CSPI) has an online guide to additives indicating whether they are safe (www.cspinet.org/reports/chemcuisine.htm). The group recommends avoiding sodium nitrite, saccharin, caffeine, olestra, acesulfame K, and artificial colourings as they are among the most questionable additives.

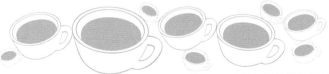

49 BAG A BOX

Look out for box schemes run by local farmers or groups of farmers. Many of them now stock a wide range of ethical and organic products – not just vegetables – and are often great sources of recipe ideas. They have the potential to transform your diet, bringing vegetables into your kitchen that you might have overlooked in the supermarket.

50 GET PLANNING

Reduce food waste and get the most out of your food by planning a series of meals which follow on from each other. For example, start with a roast chicken, and the next day use any leftover chicken in a stir-fry (making sure it is hot all the way through). The day after that use the last bits of chicken from the carcass in a stew bulked out with root vegetables. This will also help cut down the amount of meat you are buying.

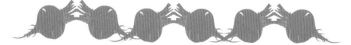

51 FARM FRESH

There are around 550 farmers' markets in the UK and about £120 million is spent at them each year. By buying directly from farmers you will be supporting local producers and ensuring the goods you buy have not travelled miles to reach you. But remember that not all products will be certified organic and you may want to check with individual stallholders about the sustainability of their products.

52 SAVE MONEY AT THE MARKET

County and local markets also offer a good source of fresh fruit and vegetables – often fresher than the produce you'll find in supermarkets with their ability to keep food in storage. Plus, you'll be saving some money at the market. Fruit and vegetables sold in supermarkets are around 30% more expensive than those available from street markets, according to UK pressure group Sustain.

53 GET PICKING

Look out for local 'pick your own' farms and orchards. You'll be doing some exercise in the great outdoors, getting to know your local farmers and educating your children about the way in which food is grown. Plus, you can be confident in the freshness of your food. Look online for sites near you or check out www.pickyourown.org which lists farms internationally.

54 DOWN ON THE FARM

Many farms now have shops, in fact, there are an estimated 4,000 of them in the UK, and they are great sources of locally produced foods. They often include traditional butchers and cheese-makers, plus you'll frequently find breeds of livestock and varieties of fruit and vegetables that supermarkets overlook. You'll be reducing food miles and getting more diversity in your diet.

55 THE AIR DEBATE

Aircraft emissions produce far more greenhouse gases per 'food mile' than any other form of transport – in the UK, less than 1% of imported food is air freighted but it contributes 11% of the carbon emissions from food distribution. But, dropping all air-freighted food from your shopping list could be disastrous for fragile farming communities in the developing world. UK certifier the Soil Association may offer a solution to the dilemma – it is considering only certifying air freighted organic food if it meets its own Ethical Trade standards or similar standards and companies will have to develop plans for reducing air freight.

56 GO WILD IN THE WILD

Look out for nutritious wild foods in your neighbourhood, whether in your garden, hedgerows, or in a local park or woodland. Your bounty could range from blackberries to wild garlic and mushrooms but check that the plants you pick are safe to eat, are not rare or protected species, and are not treated with chemicals.

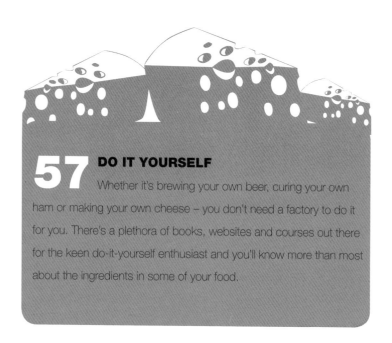

57 DO IT YOURSELF

Whether it's brewing your own beer, curing your own ham or making your own cheese – you don't need a factory to do it for you. There's a plethora of books, websites and courses out there for the keen do-it-yourself enthusiast and you'll know more than most about the ingredients in some of your food.

58 ALL THAT REMAINS

Peelings from your vegetables, the remains of a roast, or washed trimmings … all of these can be used to make a mineral-rich stock which is itself a part of many other dishes such soups. It saves on food waste and will help you to avoid processed stock cubes or powders, many of which contain flavour enhancers and loads of salt.

59 GET ON THE LEARNING CURVE

The boom in demand for organic food and the popularity of the slow food movement show that there is a growing interest in natural and eco-friendly food. And all this interest means there's no shortage of courses out there to improve your knowledge – from residential wild food courses to cheese-making and beekeeping courses. See www.lowimpact.org/courses.htm for courses and www.slowfood.com for further education and events.

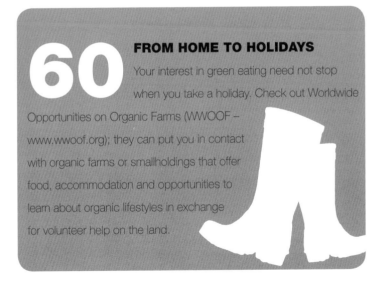

60 FROM HOME TO HOLIDAYS

Your interest in green eating need not stop when you take a holiday. Check out Worldwide Opportunities on Organic Farms (WWOOF – www.wwoof.org); they can put you in contact with organic farms or smallholdings that offer food, accommodation and opportunities to learn about organic lifestyles in exchange for volunteer help on the land.

61 DITCH THE FLAVOURINGS

There are around 2,700 different flavourings currently allowed in our food but they do not need to be identified, so it is impossible to know exactly what is being added to our food and drink and how much of them we consume, according to the Food Commission. These flavourings have no nutritional value and often they replace genuine, nutritious ingredients – fooling us into believing that a fat-, sugar- or salt-laden food is in fact a fruit-based healthy option.

62 IS IT REALLY NATURAL?

Don't be fooled by the term 'natural flavourings'. While the flavouring should have come from a 'natural' vegetable, animal or microbiological source, an apple flavour doesn't necessarily have to come from an apple. In fact, natural flavourings can originate from unexpected 'natural' sources, such as carcasses and oak wood chips. And even when the flavour has come from apples, the goodness will be lost in the production process.

63 GO EASY ON THE SALT

Too much salt raises your blood pressure and thus increases your risk of heart disease and stroke so it's best to cut back. But avoiding salt can be tough – 75% of the salt we eat is already in the food we buy, such as breakfast cereals, sauces, soups and ready-meals, according to the Food Standards Agency. The best tip is to read the label and avoid processed foods in the first place, with the additional benefit of saving on the packaging and carbon emissions associated with these foods.

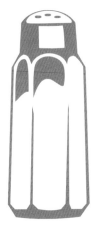

64 SALT OF THE SEA

Consider buying unrefined natural sea salt. It's higher in minerals and trace elements that are lost in the processing of table salt, and as it has a better flavour, less is needed in your food. Choose ones that have been harvested using sustainable techniques and avoid all salts with anti-caking agents.

65 IS IT SO SWEET?

Most people in the developing world are eating too much sugar – it is rotting our teeth and contributing to the obesity epidemic. But it isn't just our health that is suffering. A WWF report shows that sugar may be responsible for more biodiversity loss than any other crop. Cut back the amount you eat by avoiding cakes and biscuits, and drinking fewer sugary, fizzy drinks.

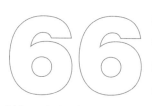

SWEET BAKING

When buying sugar for home baking, choose those that are certified as both organic and fairly traded to be sure that the environment and those working with the sugar are being protected from exploitation. Opt for unrefined raw cane sugar as this will not have been refined using chemicals and bleaching agents – even 'brown' sugar is just refined white sugar that has been coloured with caramel or raw cane molasses.

67

LOW-CAL CAUTION

For those seeking to reduce their calorie intake without giving up sweet treats, artificial sweeteners appear to be the answer. But while they may be more or less calorie-free, they involve carbon-hungry manufacturing processes and are full of chemicals that are linked to possible health risks. Artificial sweeteners are not allowed in organic food.

68

A TRADITIONAL LOAF

Almost all of the bread industrial bakers sell is made with enzymes. These don't have to be declared as an ingredient as they are deemed to be a 'processing aid' and there is currently no safety evaluation of food enzymes at European level, but there are concerns that they could cause allergies. Find a traditional artisan baker and ask how they make their bread.

69 FAT IN YOUR BREAD

Of the 9 million loaves of bread eaten each day in the UK most will come from vast industrial bakeries where vegetable fat is used to keep the loaf fresher for longer. Not only is this more saturated fat that your body could do without, it could also be at the expense of the world's great forests. Millions of hectares of tropical rainforest are being cleared yearly for the planting of palm oil crops and it is often palm oil that is being used in bread.

70 BAKE BREAD

Go back to a simpler time when bread was made of flour, salt, water and yeast – bake your own. There are many recipes available and plenty of advice online. You will be able to avoid additives and preservatives such as sodium stearoyl lactylate and diglycerides so common in shop-bought breads, as well as feel empowered by creating nutritious and delicious food from the wholesome ingredients you have chosen. For more on why it's worth the effort see www.breadmatters.com.

71

DO YOU KNEAD IT?

Unfortunately, far too many people think the first step to baking bread is a dash to their nearest electrical store to buy a bread- maker. But over the past ten years electricity consumption from consumer electronics and domestic computers in the UK has increased by 47% and is expected to rise by 82% by 2011. Cut back on your power consumption and get kneading – it will be good for toning your arms as well – but start with a simple recipe first.

72

CATERERS WHO CARE

If you are a regular user of caterers then it's time to review your sourcing. Look out for the new breed of eco-catering companies which specialize in organic, eco-friendly food and will be able to put together nutritionally balanced menus as well.

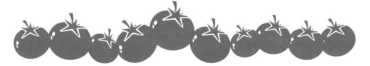

73 GASTRONOMICALLY GREEN

A growing number of restaurants are starting to take responsibility for the planet, and in London they have formed a network called Ethical Eats. For example, the Acorn House restaurant in London has a green roof for growing the herbs used in their dishes and their own water-purification system. The reason it matters? Recent research found that the CO_2 produced by a selection of restaurant meals in London, based on imported ingredients from non-European countries, is on average more than a hundred times higher than that of ingredients produced in Britain.

74 CERTIFIED GREEN

In the US, a Green Restaurant Association has been established since 1990 to help restaurants become more environmentally sustainable. Check out its Certified Green Restaurant Guide which lists those that meet its standards at www.dinegreen.com.

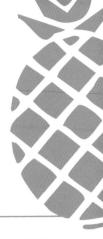

75

CAFÉ CULTURE

Many local cafés are still bastions of deep-fried food but there are healthier alternatives. Juice bars are great options for healthy salads and fresh-pressed drinks, or choose vegan or vegetarian cafés. Some specialty restaurants, such as VitaOrganic in London, focus on raw foods and food cooked at a low temperature to optimize vitamin content.

76

ALL BAR NONE

The refreshments on offer in most pubs and bars aren't known for their health-giving properties but some places are trying to change all that. Look out for organic 'gastropubs' that offer seasonal, organic, locally sourced food along with locally brewed beers and organic wines and spirits.

77

FISH FACTS

Atlantic cod stocks are currently at historic low levels and the species is now threatened with commercial extinction in UK waters. Only buy cod that has been line-caught from a sustainable fishery or choose alternatives such as rock salmon. Cod, hake, halibut and plaice are usually caught by bottom trawling, which destroys the seabed.

78

FISHY FARE

Many restaurants are starting to realize that customers care about the sustainability of their food and this includes the fish on the menu. Look out for those that include details of how the fish is caught (always opt for line-caught fish) and seek out restaurants that carry the Marine Stewardship Council (MSC) eco-label.

79

WHERE'S THE INFO?

Fast food is often high in fat, additives, sugar and salt, but you'd be hard-pressed to find out just how high.

A recent National Consumer Council study in the UK has found that leading takeaway chains still offer little, if any, nutritional information to help customers make healthy choices. Buy food from somewhere that is happy to shout about the nutritional content of its meals.

80

NOT SO FAST

Britons eat almost 2 billion takeaway meals a year while in the US nearly half the money spent on food goes on food prepared away from home. But while many fast-food chains are making improvements to their menus and practices, as with supermarkets, the scale and the way they operate means they are never going to be the best eco-friendly option.

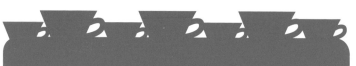

81 USE YOUR OWN CUP

The fast-food industry giants such as Wendy's and McDonald's are some of the largest consumers of paper products in the US and much of the paper is coming from the Southern forests, where many species of plant are endangered due to habitat loss. Next time you want a coffee take your own cup along and say no to napkins and cup holders. See nofreerefills.org for more ideas.

82 A MEATY MATTER

Eat less meat. A report for the United Nations, 'Livestock's Long Shadow', has found that the meat industry is responsible for 18% of greenhouse gases – more than all forms of transport put together – and leads to deforestation, acid rain and desertification. According to Environmental Defense, if every American skipped one meal of chicken per week and substituted vegetarian foods instead, the carbon dioxide savings would be the same as taking more than a half-million cars off US roads.

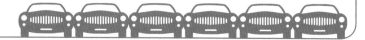

83 FEED THE HUNGRY

Raising livestock uses a disproportionate amount of the world's resources which could be better employed in feeding the hungry. For example, in the US it is estimated that 70% of all grains, 80% of all agricultural land, half of all water resources, and one-third of all fossil fuels are used to raise animals for food. When you hear about global food shortages, ponder the fact that there is already enough grain grown on earth to feed 10 billion vegetarian people but much of it is fed to cattle.

84 DON'T SEE RED

Red meat is a rich source of protein, iron, vitamin B12 and zinc, but some clear links are emerging between the consumption of red meat and certain diseases such as bowel cancer. By cutting back on red meat you will doing your body a favour and helping the environment – the world's 1.5 billion cattle are among the greatest threat to the climate, forests and wildlife.

GO FOR GRASS

Producing red meat really does cost this planet dear – for example, scientists have found that producing 1 kg (2.2 lb) of beef results in the same CO_2 emissions that would be released by European car every 250 kilometres (155 miles) and the energy consumption is equal to a 100-watt bulb being left on for 20 days. But in 2003, a Swedish study found that raising organic beef on grass, rather than feed, reduced greenhouse gas emissions by 40% and consumed 85% less energy.

A QUESTION OF BREEDING

If you decide to have a meat treat then go for local traditional breeds such as Sussex cattle, one of the oldest English breeds. You will be doing your bit to support biodiversity, reducing food miles (especially if the meat came via a local abattoir) and traditional breeds are often farmed less intensively.

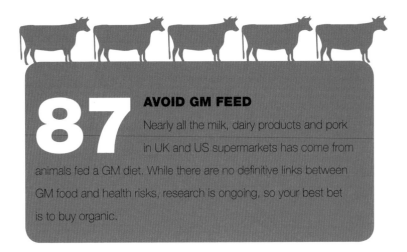

87 AVOID GM FEED

Nearly all the milk, dairy products and pork in UK and US supermarkets has come from animals fed a GM diet. While there are no definitive links between GM food and health risks, research is ongoing, so your best bet is to buy organic.

88 CHEAP ISSUES

Don't be tempted by cheap meat. To produce beef, pork and poultry in large quantities cheaply, industrial farmers cut corners that harm the environment and result in a lower quality of meat. Most intensively-reared animals are given antibiotics daily, and this use has been linked to the rise of antibiotic-resistant superbugs such as the *Staphylococcus aureus* bacterium, MRSA. In the US, beef is commonly injected with hormones to increase their growth rate (see also tip 113).

89 A GOOD LIFE

Treating animals well brings benefits for you, too. For example, studies have shown that factory-farmed chickens contain more fat and less iron than traditional breeds of chicken that are usually farmed in free-range or organic conditions, with ample space to roam. Intensively farmed chickens are given high-energy foods and are inactive, so a typical supermarket chicken in the West contains more fat than protein, with 2.7 times as much fat as in 1970.

90 BEWARE WASHED CHICKEN IMPORTS

The US chicken industry widely uses antimicrobial washes for poultry meat but there are concerns that this masks the underlying cause of bacterial contamination in the first place and could lead to further antibiotic resistance in humans. The EU banned antimicrobial washes for poultry meat in 1997 but there is pressure to lift the ban in order to allow trade. Find out if the chicken you've been buying has been washed.

91 GO FOR GRASS

Look for beef from cattle fed grass-based diets as American research has found it has up to 500% more of two types of conjugated linoleic acids (CLAs) than beef from animals fed high cereal-maize diets. These CLAs are believed to protect against cancer, and red meat and milk from grass-fed animals are the richest dietary sources. All organic cattle in the EU have grass-based diets.

92 LAMB CHOICES

Sheep don't lend themselves to intensive farming, so whether you buy organic or not, your lamb is likely to have been naturally produced with sheep grazing freely in open countryside. Organic sheep feed mostly on pesticide-free grass will have received far fewer veterinary treatments than non-organic sheep. Soil Association organic standards ban the use of organophosphorus sheep dips to control infestation as they have serious health implications for animals and humans.

93 UPLAND ISSUES

In the UK, almost two-thirds of sheep are in hill and upland areas but overstocking and overgrazing have caused widespread ecological damage; this leads to barren landscapes that can no longer absorb all the rain that falls, increasing the risk of flooding in towns and cities. But a recent change in agricultural subsidies is seeing a decline in hill farming which is resulting in too little grazing and therefore a loss of habitat for some birds. Support hill farmers that are managing the land sustainably.

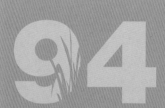

94 DIP INTO A DIRECTORY

Help is at hand if you want to get the health benefits of grass-fed meat. In the US and Canada Eatwild's Directory of Farms has a listing of more than 800 pasture-based farms (www.eatwild.com) while in the UK, Seeds of Health lists grass-fed meat producers (www.seedsofhealth.co.uk).

95 PICK ECOLOGICAL

It doesn't have to be organic to be an ecological option. These days you can pick from a variety of meat and cheeses that have come from sheep and cattle grazed on biodiverse pastures, such as moorland and salt marshes, rich in wild plant species. Research has shown that not only does this kind of grazing assist the biodiversity of the sites, there are also health and taste benefits for the consumer. Look online for suppliers.

96 CUT BACK ON PROCESSED MEAT

Researchers from the US National Cancer Institute found that both red and processed meats increased risks for bowel and lung cancer, and between them raised the risk of developing other cancers such as throat cancer and pancreatic cancer (in men). In the case of processed meat, there are concerns that additive sodium nitrite – used as a preservative and to fix the colour of the meat – is carcinogenic.

97 V IS FOR VENISON

Venison might be a more eco-friendly red meat option than beef since there are a number of small, sustainable providers of wild venison who are actually helping to protect endangered species, such as bluebells, that are under threat from a recent rise in the number of deer. Like most red meat, it is a good source of protein and iron but as a bonus it is fairly low in fat, including saturated fat.

98 ALL IN AN EGG

Eggs contain 13 essential vitamins and minerals, are a good source of high-quality protein and are rich in antioxidants. But buy your eggs from pasture-raised chickens which have been allowed to roam freely. Numerous studies have found that eggs from poultry raised on pasture have been shown to have higher levels of vitamins A, B12 and E and far higher amounts of omega-3 fatty acids than conventional eggs. Plus, it uses less energy as there is no need to transport feed and animal waste.

99

BATTERIES ARE BAD

Battery cages give laying hens less space than a sheet of paper. As well as leading to psychological and physical suffering for hens, recent scientific research has found that battery eggs are more likely to carry salmonella than free-range or organic eggs. Europe is banning the use of battery cages by 2012 but currently more than 75% of European hens are kept in them, while in the US nearly 280 million laying hens are confined in cages (according to the Humane Society).

100

RAISE YOUR OWN

If you want to be certain that your eggs come from happy, healthy, truly free-range chickens, then consider keeping your own, but check with your local regulating body whether you need permission. Try www.mypetchicken.com for advice, and remember to feed them your food scraps and use their manure on your compost.

101

BREAST IS BEST

There is no doubt that breast milk is the most complete nutritional option available to babies, helping protect them against a myriad of infections in the early years while also providing a range of nutrients that formula milks still aren't able to match. But think too of all those plastic bottles and teats, the packets of formula and the energy used to sterilize …breast is best for the planet, too.

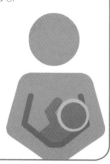

102

JUNK THE JUNK

A British study has found that eating a diet of fatty, processed food when pregnant or breastfeeding may result in children with high levels of fat in their bloodstream and fat around the major organs, potentially leading to the development of type II diabetes and heart disease in the future.

103

AVOID SOYA FORMULA

With growing demand for soya leading to deforestation around the world it is a good idea to avoid soya-based formula milk but there are other good reasons for this too. There are concerns that it could affect babies' reproductive development due to the high levels of plant hormones or phytoestrogens in soya.

104

HONEY FOR YOUR HONEY

You might think that sweetening baby food with a natural product like local honey rather than imported refined sugar is both better for the baby and the planet but it is actually a bad idea for any child under one. It is rare, but honey can contain a bacterium that causes infant botulism so wait until they are over one (and remember, honey is still a type of sugar so use sparingly).

105 PUREE POWER

The best introduction to nutritious and eco-friendly eating habits for babies is homemade baby food. You can be sure that the food you give them is fresh, made from organic ingredients with no pesticide residues and doesn't contain additives. Cook in bulk, purée in a blender and freeze in ice-cube trays – simple.

106 SNACK ATTACK

Encouraging children to snack on fresh fruit will not only help their health, it will help cut down on the packaging mountain that comes from crisp packets, sweet wrappers and so on. Given that around seven out of ten items of litter are food related, this should also help reduce the waste on our streets, beaches and green spaces.

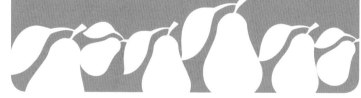

107 DIY CRISPS

A 35 g (1.2 oz) single-portion bag of crisps (potato chips) contains two-and-a-half teaspoons of oil, and is also three times as salty as sea water – containing half the recommended daily salt intake for a six-year-old. Choose versions made with unpeeled potatoes, as these will have a higher fibre content. Best of all, make your own from root vegetables, such as parsnips or beetroot.

108 PACK LIGHT

All too often, packed lunches are heavy on waste packaging and light on nutrition. Make them a lesson in green and healthy living by using reusable containers, ditching the individually wrapped items and learning about healthy options. There are lots of ideas online – see www.wastefreelunches.org and www.schoolfoodtrust.org.uk.

109

A LOT OF BOTTLE

Britons now consume about 85m litres (180m pints) of milk a week, at least two-thirds of which is sold by supermarkets in plastic bottles, which either end up in landfill or are shipped hundreds of miles for recycling, mostly in China. Find and support a local milk delivery service – they often use electric vehicles and will pick-up and re-use the bottles. Look online at www.findmeamilkman.net or www.winderfarms.com/homedelivery/milkmenacrossamerica.

110

MILK IT

European research has found that organic milk has nearly 70% more essential fatty acid omega-3 than its non-organic equivalent and other studies have also shown organic milk contains significantly more vitamin E and beta-carotene. This is likely to be due to the cows' diet – organic cows graze freely on fresh grass and clover while most non-organic cows eat a more grain-based diet.

111 CONSIDER UHT

It could be greener to buy UHT (Ultra High Temperature) milk – milk that has been heated to a higher temperature than pasteurized milk – as it doesn't require storing in large energy-guzzling refrigerators. UHT milk is popular in Europe, accounting for over 90% of milk consumption in France, Spain and Belgium, but in Britain it makes up only 8.4% of the milk market. In the US, Parmalat UHT milk is sold, and many food products are made using UHT milk.

112 A BAG OF MILK, PLEASE

In Canada, 40% of milk is delivered in bags and now British consumers are getting the same opportunity. The bags, or packs, use 75% less plastic than a standard one-litre plastic milk bottle. You buy a jug to keep in the fridge and top it up with the bags. The idea is to stop 100,000 plastic milk bottles hitting our landfill sites each year. But in order to offset the energy used to make the non-recyclable jug you need to keep using it.

113 HORMONE-FREE

In the US, cows are commonly injected with an artificial, genetically engineered growth hormone (rBGH) in order to increase the per-cow milk yield. But these hormones have been linked to increasing risks of developing breast and colon cancers. Milk from hormone-treated cows doesn't have to be labelled so look for milk labelled 'No rBGH' or check online for a list of those hormone-free milk producers (www.organicconsumers.org/rBGH/rbghlist.cfm).

114 EAT YOUR CHEESE

There are around 700 cheeses produced in Britain alone, but they account for only 65% of the cheese eaten in the UK. Instead of driving up demand for imported food, seek out local cheese makers and support their businesses. Goat's and ewe's milk cheeses are likely to have the lowest carbon emissions since cows have a bigger carbon footprint. You could also try making your own – www.cheesemaking.co.uk has advice on how to get started.

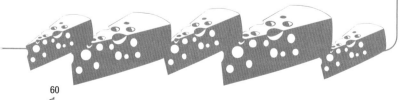

115 AN APPLE A DAY

A non-organic apple can be sprayed up to 16 times with 36 different chemicals, many of which cannot simply be washed off. British government tests, carried out in 2005, found pesticides in 80% of non-organic apple samples. Choose organic to cut out chemicals in your diet or research pesticides used on fruit at www.pesticides.gov.uk or www.epa.gov/pesticides/about/types.htm.

116 PEEL ALERT

According to the WWF, orange production requires more intensive use of pesticides than any other major crops. If pesticide residues do remain on the fruit (and in 2007 the British Pesticides Residues Committee found residues from more than one pesticide on all 37 samples of soft citrus fruits tested) then they are likely to be on the peel. So avoid using non-organic peel in your recipes and buy organic marmalade.

117 PICK YOUR VEGETABLES

Help is at hand when it comes to finding out which vegetables are in season. The website www.thinkvegetables.co.uk lists those that are in season in the UK and ranks veggies according to their value in terms of particular vitamins or phytochemicals. In the US search www.sustainabletable.org/shop/eatseasonal for a state-by-state directory of crops in season.

118 GROW IT, DON'T BUY IT

Cultivate your own vegetables and fruit without using pesticides and herbicides and you will know that your food is as fresh and natural as possible. From a selection of herbs on your windowsill to a raised bed filled with tomatoes, strawberries and runner beans – you can grow at the scale that suits you.

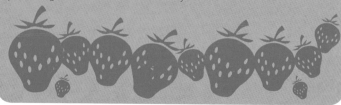

119 BUCK THE TREND

Just a few varieties of fruits and vegetables are grown and sold commercially, chosen by supermarkets and their suppliers for regularity of shape, colour and flawless appearance, rather than flavour or continuity. This has led to the loss of many tasty, nutrition-packed varieties, which is bad for biodiversity and potentially leaves us exposed to future pests and diseases. So look for unusual varieties, support retailers that are bucking the trend and plant your own heritage seeds.

120 EAT YOUR WEEDS

Don't overlook the green stuff in your garden, even if they are just weeds. Some weeds make tasty additions to salads, so give nettles, dandelion, purslane and lamb's quarters (*chenopodium album*, also known as wild spinach) a try when the plants are young and tender. You'll find more information and recipes online.

121 ADOPT A VEGETABLE

You can do more to keep some wonderful old varieties of vegetables alive than growing them. Britain's organic growing charity, Garden Organic, looks after over 800 varieties of rare and heirloom vegetables in its Heritage Seed Library, and is offering people the chance to 'Adopt a Veg' (www.gardenorganic.org.uk), which conserves a variety by paying for the seed handling, storage and propagation facilities.

122 GET SPROUTING

You don't need much space to grow your own nutrition-packed sprouts. Use on old jar or invest in a sprouter, buy organic, non-GM sprout seeds (try your local health food store for these) and off you go (remembering to soak and rinse them first). They could be ready to eat in as little as 12 hours for quinoa and five to six days for most others.

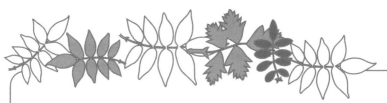

123 HERBY HOMES

As well as fruit and vegetables, be sure to grow some herbs – if only on a windowsill. Chives, mint, basil, parsley – start with those you use regularly and experience the thrill of snipping minutes before eating. It'll also save you buying costly vacuum-packed, pesticide-laden herbs that have been flown in to a supermarket near you.

124 GROW IN A GROUP

Whether it's in local allotments, a disused area of public space or in school grounds, community food-growing clubs are thriving around the world – not only providing fresh local produce but also teaching children about food and nutrition. If you are keen to set up a school food-growing project, check out www.growinggrub.co.uk and www.growingcommunities.org.uk. In the US contact the National Garden Club at www.gardenclub.org.

125

FROZEN IN TIME

Frozen vegetables are usually processed within a few hours of harvest and there is little nutrient loss in the freezing process so frozen vegetables are likely to have a higher vitamin and mineral content than some fresh vegetables, which often take days or weeks to reach the dinner table.

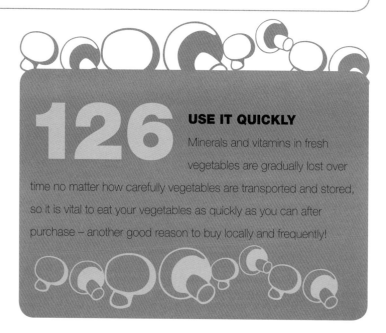

126

USE IT QUICKLY

Minerals and vitamins in fresh vegetables are gradually lost over time no matter how carefully vegetables are transported and stored, so it is vital to eat your vegetables as quickly as you can after purchase – another good reason to buy locally and frequently!

127

GO RAW

By eating a lot of raw fruit and vegetables you will be saving power, have fewer pans to go in the dishwasher, and be doing your health the world of good by reducing the amount of cooked, processed or highly refined foods in your diet.

128

GIVE IT A SCRUB

Wash your fruit and vegetables, especially if you don't buy organic, since your produce is likely to have been sprayed with pesticides or other chemicals. A good scrub will help remove some of these, although be aware that many agricultural chemicals are trapped under a wax coating added to resist water and prolong shelf life. There are several products out there that can help, such as Organiclean or Veggie-Wash, or you can try soaking produce for five minutes in a 50/50 solution of white vinegar and water. But remember to always fill a bowl with water rather than to wash produce under a running tap (faucet).

129 DON'T SEEK PERFECTION

Bent carrots, odd shaped spuds ... nature doesn't go in for standardization. Yet, every year thousands of tonnes of perfectly tasty fruit and vegetables are thrown away by supermarkets because they don't look good. The retailers say their customers won't buy any produce that is less than perfect ... prove them wrong!

130 PESTICIDE PERIL

Up to 40% of the fruit, vegetable and bread samples tested in the UK were found to contain pesticides albeit at 'safe' levels, while in the US, consumers can experience up to 70 daily exposures to residues through their diets. Given that more than 300 man-made chemicals have been found in human bodies, the best way to avoid chemical contact from your fruit and veg is to eat certified organic foods.

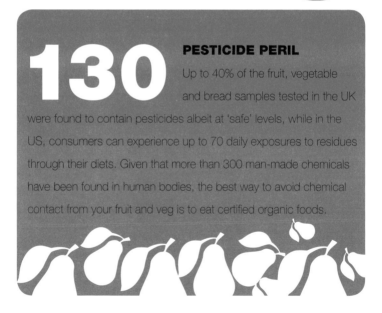

131 SURPRISE BENEFITS

You may be routinely throwing away beneficial parts of your vegetables. Take the leafy tops on beetroot for example, or salad onion leaves. Before cutting and binning take a look online for recipes and cooking tips; you may be surprised to see what you could have been eating for all these years. But don't be tempted to give rhubarb leaves a try – these really are very poisonous when eaten raw or cooked.

132 SALAD DAYS

If you are a sucker for those pre-washed and bagged salad leaves in the supermarket, then stop and think again. According to the World Wide Fund for Nature (WWF), they are often immersed in chlorine at concentrations up to twenty times higher than the average swimming pool. Dump the plastic bags of leaves and give growing your own a try – salad leaves are incredibly easy and fun to produce.

133 DRESS IT WELL

It's a health crime to make a beautiful salad using organic leaves, sprouts, veggies or fruits and then smother it in a highly processed, unhealthy dressing. Make your own using just a few ingredients – you can get away with just one part vinegar to two parts good quality olive oil, with a dash of mustard or garlic for taste – and experiment with flavours.

134 GET WITH THE BEET

Don't overlook traditional, seasonal vegetables such as the humble beetroot. It is one of the best dietary sources of folate and is a good source of vitamin C, potassium, manganese and fibre. Deep red varieties are rich in anthocyanins, which may reduce cancer risk and you can also eat beetroot's green leaves, which contain betacarotene, calcium and iron.

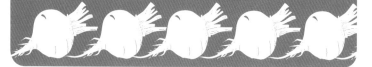

135 MUSHROOM MAGIC

You can grow your very own mushrooms by purchasing a mushroom-growing kit. The easiest culinary mushrooms to grow at home are oyster, shiitake, wine cap and portobello, but many more possibilities exist. Mushrooms are low in salt and fat and provide dietary fibre, some protein and significant quantities of B vitamins. They are also good source of minerals, including iron.

136 TIME FOR SOME SPUDS

Britons eat 94 kg (207 lb) of potatoes each a year – and for good reason; they are packed with potassium, iron and other nutrients such as vitamins C, B6 and B1. In fact, one portion of spuds can provide 19% of the recommended daily intake of iron compared with pasta's 7%. Rather than flying your pasta in from overseas, pick some potatoes for your next meal and support local farmers.

137 LOCAL CARROTS

Carrots are Britain's second most popular vegetable after potatoes and almost all of the carrots we buy are grown in the UK, but there are still issues relating to food miles. According to Sustain, carrots, like other food, are travelling nearly 60% further on the UK roads than in the 1970s due to the centralization of food distribution. Buy your carrots loose from local, preferably organic growers.

138 PEEL IT

Pesticide use on carrots has been such a matter of health concern that the British government actually advises consumers to peel and top carrots before eating, which will remove about four-fifths of the residue – unfortunately it also removes nutrients in the peel. This is just another good reason to buy organic!

139

GET A GROWBAG

Tomatoes are taking a heavy toll on our environment. The World Wildlife Fund says that tomato production uses high levels of agro-chemicals, such as methyl bromide for disinfecting soil, damages and pollutes rivers and causes soil erosion. They are another easy crop to grow for anyone with a small amount of space in a sunny spot and you can buy organic growbags to make life really easy.

140

GO BANANAS

It's official … bananas are the world's most popular fruit with almost 5 billion US dollars' worth sold each year. But the banana business has caused widespread deforestation, the pollution of coral reefs and waterways, and contamination from toxic agrochemicals. It also has a history of exploitation when it comes to paying a fair price to growers. Look for organic, fairtrade or Rainforest Alliance certified bananas.

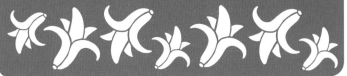

141 BERRIES FROM HEAVEN

The superfruit trend has seen a soaring demand for products like goji berries (which come from a vine that grows in China, Tibet and other areas of Asia) and the Brazilian palm tree super-berry acai, based on their high nutritional value. But while they may be high in vitamins and antioxidants, so are many other fruits grown nearer to home.

142 SUPPORT FOR ORCHARDS

Since 1970, over 60% of UK apple orchards have been lost and, although there are around 6,000 varieties of dessert and cooking apples and hundreds more cider apples, today just 10 types of apple account for 92% of the UK's area of eating apple orchards. In the US, only 15 varieties account for 90% of total production. Seek out traditional or 'heirloom' varieties, and look out too for unusual varieties of damson, plums, cherries and pears. Heirloom apple farms will often sell cuttings from their trees as well as the fruit.

143

CHEERS TO CHERRIES

Cherry orchards are going the same way as apple orchards in the UK – in 50 years 90% of cherry orchards have been lost and 95% of cherries eaten in the nation are now imported. Benefit from a better local supply of this healthy fruit by supporting Cherry Aid, and even renting your own cherry tree for a year (see www. foodloversbritain.com).

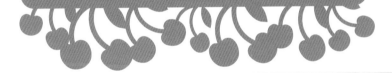

144

DRIED FRUIT DANGERS

Dried fruit is full of fibre and vitamins but there are some health fears linked to the use of sulphur dioxide as a dried fruit preservative. Ten years ago the World Health Organization (WHO) warned that up to 20–30% of childhood asthmatics may be sensitive to sulphite preservatives and recommended their use be reduced or phased out. Seek out organic non-sulphured apricots and avoid the many over-packaged dried fruit snack products for children.

145 COOK IN BULK

Prepare more than you need of your favourite dishes and freeze the excess. You will be saving energy and will be far less likely to reach for an over-packaged, processed ready meal when you are next short of time – you'll have your own stock of healthy dinners in the freezer.

146 GREEN STEAM

Steaming your vegetables and fish will minimize nutrient loss, especially vitamin C, vitamin B1 and mineral salts. For example, a study has found that when steaming fresh broccoli 11% of flavonoids were lost compared to 47% lost when pressure cooked, 66% lost when boiled and 97% lost when microwaved. Plus, if you use a layered steamer, it will ensure you make the most of the energy used to cook your food.

147

UNDER PRESSURE

Although using a pressure cooker does result in more nutrient loss than steaming, it is still better than boiling or microwaving your food, and as it cooks three or four times more quickly than a conventional cooker, it will save energy.

148

HOB OF CHOICE

A gas hob is considered more energy efficient than electric, with the exception of induction hobs. They are more expensive than traditional hobs, but consume half as much electricity as electric hobs and are more efficient in heat transfer. Manufacturers estimate that power savings of 40–70% are achievable.

149

USE LESS WATER

Valuable nutrients, such as the water-soluble B vitamins and vitamin C, can be lost by using too much water when preparing and cooking your fruit and vegetables, and of course we are all being asked to save as much water as possible. So instead of soaking your produce, just give it a quick rinse, use less water when boiling or microwaving and cook until just crisp.

150

KEEP A LID ON IT

If you are boiling food then make sure you keep a lid on your pots and pans. This will speed up the cooking time and allow you to use less water, which also benefits the nutritional content of your food.

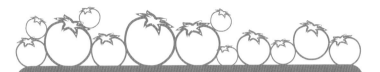

151

AVOID ALUMINIUM

According to the Food Standards Agency in the UK, it's best not to use aluminium pans, baking trays and foil, or other cookware made of aluminium to cook foods that are highly acidic, such as tomatoes, rhubarb, cabbage and many soft fruits. A study has found that about 20% of the aluminium in our diet comes from aluminium cookware and foil.

152

STIR-FRY TO GET YOUR VEG

Fried food is invariably high in fat and best avoided; however, stir-frying food over a high heat for a short period of time and using minimal oil will not result in a fatty dish and can be a good way to eat more vegetables, along with other traditional, healthy stir-fry ingredients such as ginger, garlic and tofu.

153 GIVE IT A SPRAY

Use a hand-pump oil spray if you need to fry food and especially when browning meat and vegetables. Spray the pan lightly and you will reduce the amount of oil absorbed by the food, and ultimately reduce the volume of oil you need to buy.

154 DON'T PEEL

If you buy organic fruit and vegetables, then peeling is mostly unnecessary from a health perspective and could reduce the nutritional value of your food. Rather than waste a vitamin- and fibre-rich part of your diet, keep the peel on and just give it a quick scrub in a little water. For those items which need peeling, a banana or orange say, then make sure the peelings go on a compost heap and not in the garbage bin.

155 BE ADVENTUROUS

You don't just have to stick with brown rice and oatmeal – there's a whole world of healthy grains out there, including amaranth, emmer, farro, grano (lightly pearled wheat), spelt, triticale, bulgur (cracked wheat), millet, quinoa and sorghum. But always opt for organic and support local farmers where possible.

156 WHEAT CONCERNS

More land is used to grow wheat than any other crop in the world, which is why the way in which it is grown matters so much for biodiversity. Unfortunately, conventional wheat farming uses large amounts of artificial fertilizers, is a big user of chemicals such as herbicides, soil fumigants, insecticides and fungicides, and demands a lot of water – it is the second most irrigated crop globally.

157 CUT BACK ON RICE

More than 90% of the world's rice harvest is grown and consumed in Asia, which means that unless you live there your rice has probably notched up quite a few food miles. It is also likely that it will have been treated with chemicals – Asian rice growers use 13% of global pesticides, according to the WWF – and a great deal of water (it takes 3,000–5,000 litres of water [800–1300 gallons] to produce 1 kg [2.2 lb] of rice).

158 LOOK FOR LOCAL GRAINS

To cut your food miles and ensure you are getting a good mix of foods, look into locally produced, ideally organic, grains – likely to be oats, barley and rye for those living in northern Europe. Buy wholegrains to ensure the least amount of energy has been used in their production and to maximize nutritional content.

159 GO GLASS

When storing food choose glass containers instead of plastic. Plastic is a petroleum-based product, results in a great deal of pollution from its creation to disposal and there are concerns that freezing or heating plastic can release toxic carcinogens. If you must buy plastic containers, look for a '1' or '2' inside the recycled arrow symbol on the package as these containers are more likely to be accepted for recycling.

160 DEGRADABLE DOUBTS

You may think that the greenest packaging for your fruit and veg is the latest kind of degradable plastic, but it is causing a number of concerns. Some types require light to degrade, so if they end up buried in a landfill site they won't break down, while others that biodegrade may cause an increase in the greenhouse gas methane if they end up in landfill as opposed to a hot compost heap.

161

SORT IT OUT

It's great to recycle but make sure you do it properly or it could be a waste of everybody's efforts. Don't include plastics that can't be recycled locally – in Britain this includes margarine tubs and yoghurt pots – and wash all items thoroughly to avoid contamination. Lastly, don't mix the new breed of degradable plastics in with your recycling.

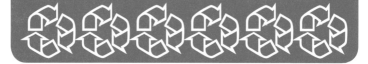

162

FRIDGE FRESH

In most households, the fridge is the single biggest energy-consuming kitchen appliance. But are you sure everything in your fridge needs chilling? Many foods need only be stored in a cool, dry place – especially if you plan to eat them reasonably quickly. It may be time to bring back the old-fashioned larder!

163 DELIGHTFUL DISHES

Hand-washing your dishes might not be the most eco-friendly option. One study has found that a dishwasher uses only half the energy and one-sixth of the water as hand-washing. Hand-washing typically uses about 63 litres (16 gallons) of water, rising to 150 litres (40 gallons) if dishes are rinsed off under running water, whereas a modern dishwasher can use just 10 litres (2 gallons) of water per cycle. But buy the most energy efficient model on the market, fill your dishwasher right up, and use phosphate-free, eco-friendly detergents.

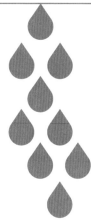

164 WRAP IT WELL

Don't wrap fatty foods, such as cheese, fried meats, pastry products and cakes with butter icing or chocolate coatings, in clingfilm (plastic wrap) since tiny amounts of chemicals can leach into these foods from the wrap. Better to choose baking paper or recycled aluminium foil, which can both be further recycled, or, in the case of the paper, added to your compost heap.

165

KEEP WELL WATERED

In the UK and US we should drink approximately 1.2 litres (6 to 8 glasses or 3 pints) of fluid every day to prevent dehydration. Ideally, this fluid should be tap water – it's better for teeth than sugary drinks, contains no calories and is free. Keep a jug of water in the fridge if you like to drink it cold, since you can waste a lot of water running the tap (faucet).

166

BAN BOTTLES

Bottled water is a cause of major environmental headaches. Empty bottles create thousands of tonnes of plastic waste – 90% of which is not recycled. Around 1.5 million barrels of oil – enough to run 100,000 cars for a year – are used to make plastic water bottles. Tap water costs a lot less and is often required to meet stringent standards.

167 FIT A FILTER

If you're unhappy with the taste of tap water or worried about its quality then it's still better to filter your water rather than buy bottled. You can fit a house water filter to your tap (faucet) and the filter will usually last up to six months, or buy a jug water filter system but look out for those with refillable cartridges, so you won't have to throw away plastic outers. Some manufacturers are also now installing recycling bins in retailers to ensure spent filters don't end up in landfill.

168 OILY ISSUES

Over 70% of all oils and fats consumed in the world come from vegetable crops – but campaign group Sustain has found that most are made by companies that do little to protect the environment or consumer health. Of particular concern are palm oil (see tip 169), olive oil (see tip 172) and rapeseed oil (see tip 171). Groundnut (peanut) and safflower oils are better choices.

169 CHECK FOR PALM OIL

Avoid food containing palm oil, which is found in one in ten supermarket products including chocolate, bread and crisps. Not only is it a saturated fat, but the growing demand for palm oil is driving the deforestation of the earth's rainforests. Check if your food retailer is buying from a sustainable source and ask if it is present in your products (it's often labelled 'vegetable oil').

170 IS BUTTER BETTER?

Butter is a less-processed product since it must be at least 80% fat and the only additive allowed is salt, whereas margarine can be mixture of oils and fats along with a range of additives; many also contain the health-harming hydrogenated vegetable oils to extend their shelf life.

171

RAPESEED ISSUES

Rapeseed oil is lower in saturated fat and has a higher vitamin E content than olive oil. But it may be not so good in other ways. It is a winter crop and part of the big switch from spring-grown crops in the UK, which has dramatically reduced farmland biodiversity such as birds, which rely on spring crops for nesting sites. Plus, it relies heavily on fertilizers so has a poor record among arable crops for leaching nitrates into waterways.

172

OLIVE HAS DOWNSIDE

Olive oil contains monounsaturated fat, which may lower cholesterol, and polyphenols which may help to ward off cancer. But intensified olive farming in the Mediterranean region 'is a major cause of one of the biggest environmental problems affecting the EU today' according to WWF. To protect the environment buy organic or from small cooperatives.

173 HEMP HELPS

Hemp seed oil is packed with healthy goodies, such as minerals, proteins and omega-3, -6 and -9, and it is said to help with eczema, asthma, heart disease and high blood pressure. It is a sustainable crop, since it requires very few agro-chemicals, is fast-growing and nearly all of the plant can be used in some way.

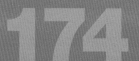

174 HYDROGENATED NIGHTMARES

One of the worst health hazards in processed foods comes from trans fats – formed when liquid oil is turned into solid fat through a process called hydrogenation. Trans fats increase the risk of coronary heart disease and are likely to have worse effects on the body than saturated fats found in butter. Both Denmark and Switzerland have banned these fats in food, but in the UK they don't even have to be listed in the ingredients. Avoid food containing hydrogenated vegetable oil.

175 BE FISH FRIENDLY

Fish, and especially oily fish, is a great option for your health. But over half of fish stocks are being fished at their maximum biological capacity and, of all the world's natural resources, fish are being depleted the fastest, according to the United Nations. So buying sustainably is imperative.

176 EAT LESS FISH

In the UK, the Food Standards Agency recommends that people should consume at least two portions of fish a week, of which one should be oily, based on its nutritional benefits. However, if 49 million adults in the UK complied with this advice it would require an extra 33 million portions of oily fish per week. Look into getting the nutrients, vitamins and oils in fish from other sources. For example, high levels of omega oils can also be found in walnuts and linseed and flax oil.

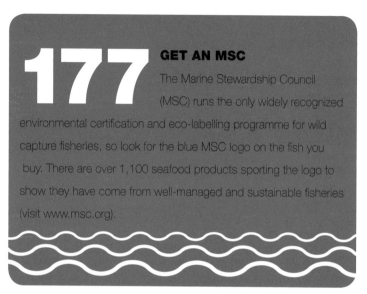

177 GET AN MSC

The Marine Stewardship Council (MSC) runs the only widely recognized environmental certification and eco-labelling programme for wild capture fisheries, so look for the blue MSC logo on the fish you buy. There are over 1,100 seafood products sporting the logo to show they have come from well-managed and sustainable fisheries (visit www.msc.org).

178 KNOWLEDGE IS POWER

Overfishing has affected oceans in every part of the world, making it a global concern. Educate yourself to be a sustainable seafood consumer. There are some great resources out there, such as the pocket fish guides from the Marine Conservation Society (www.fishonline.org), the Environmental Defense Fund (www.edf.org) and the National Audubon Society (www.seafood.audubon.org), which tell you which species to avoid eating.

179

CATCH OF THE DAY

The way your fish is caught could have cost the environment dearly. Bottom trawling can destroy sensitive marine environments while longline fishing is responsible for the death of thousands of other animals and fish caught alongside. It is estimated, for example, that 250,000 seabirds die each year because of longline fishing, including around 40,000 albatross in the Southern Ocean.

180

TUNA TIPS

Canned tuna is a good source of omega-3 fatty acids and it is hugely popular in the US. But there are health concerns regarding mercury contamination. Of the two main kinds – canned light (chunk light) and albacore tuna (solid/chunk white) – the latter averages three times the amount of mercury as that found in other canned tuna.

181 'DOLPHIN-FRIENDLY' TUNA

The term 'dolphin-friendly' on tuna labels generally means very little, according to Greenpeace, since there is no legal standard or minimum criteria applied to the term. So, while the tuna may have been fished using methods less likely to catch dolphins, it could have come from overexploited tuna stocks or have been caught using a method that has other adverse impacts. If you must buy tuna, choose line-caught skipjack tuna.

182 SUSHI SAFETY

For health and environmental reasons, steer clear of ordering sushi made with bluefin tuna. Demand from the global sushi market is driving this large fish to the brink of extinction. A recent *New York Times* report found that much of the bluefin sushi served in New York City restaurants exceeds the US FDA's 'action level' for mercury. For safe and sustainable sushi, check out the Environmental Defense Fund's Seafood Selector (www.edf.org).

183

CANNED SALMON

If you are looking for a healthy alternative to tuna, then consider opting for canned wild salmon which contains up to four times as many omega-3s as chunky light tuna, according to the USDA. The fish are usually low in contaminants but still ensure that they are sustainably caught.

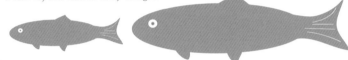

184

GO LOW ON THE FOOD CHAIN

Avoid bigger fish such as tuna, swordfish, shark and sea bass, as these accumulate toxins and heavy metals in their flesh. Opt instead for smaller 'schooling' fish such as sardines, herrings and anchovies.

185 THE COST OF SHRIMP

Shrimp fisheries have the world's highest bycatch rate – about 5 kg (11 lb) of marine life is killed for each kilo of shrimp harvested and an estimated 10 million tonnes of finfish is thrown away each year in shrimp trawl fisheries. Look instead for northern coldwater prawns that have been sustainably caught, particularly pot-caught.

186 FARMING FISH

A large amount of the fish we eat comes from fish farms – indeed in the US, over one-third of all fish eaten is farmed. But these farms can be terrible for the surrounding environment. For example, wild fish are used as feed for some farmed fish so these farm operations actually consume more fish than they produce. Other farms may pollute the surrounding ocean with faeces from the huge populations of penned fish and toxic chemicals used to kill off algae on nets.

187

SHELLFISH OPTIONS

Shellfish farms tend to be more eco-friendly than fish farms as shellfish don't need extra feed and are not concentrated in pens. Choose from farm-raised oysters, clams and mussels for a more environmentally friendly seafood option.

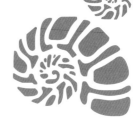

188

THE ORGANIC CHOICE

You can buy organic farmed fish from farms which will have met high environmental standards, including limits and restrictions on the use of medicines and chemicals, plus feed is sourced sustainably and stocking densities are limited. But for many, even organic farms aren't great – they can still use many of the same chemicals as conventional farmers and they still pollute the ocean with sewage – it has been estimated that an organic salmon farm can produce the same amount of untreated sewage as the population of a small town.

189 OILY BENEFITS

To get all the health benefits of oily fish without costing the environment dear, choose wild salmon from Alaska that is certified by the Marine Stewardship Council, or Scottish and Irish wild salmon. For cheaper choices try mackerel and herring.

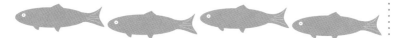

190 PRAWN PROBLEMS

Annual sales of prawns (shrimp) are growing at an average of 9% a year but this demand is driving environmental destruction around the world. Nearly 40% of world mangrove loss has been attributed to shrimp farming and mangroves are among the most productive ecosystems on the planet. If you do buy them, look out for organic or Madagascan tiger prawns as Madagascar is working towards making all its prawn fisheries sustainable.

191 SEAWEED SOLUTIONS

Seaweeds, such as kombu, wakame and nori, are becoming popular worldwide due to their nutritional and medicinal benefits. In fact, seaweeds provide all of the 56 minerals and trace minerals required by the body and contain 10 to 20 times the minerals of land plants. Buy from a company that supports traditional seaweed farming and harvesting practices and avoid hijiki – there have been concerns over high levels of the toxin arsenic found in this seaweed.

192 KEEP IT REAL WITH YOUR CEREAL

Beware the big brands and their child-friendly breakfast cereals – these products are often loaded with teeth-decaying sugar. Consumer group Which? found that out of 275 cereals tested, 52 were found to directly target children and 88% of these were found to be high in sugar. A good number of them are among the saltiest of children's foods. Look for healthier options that are GM-, sugar- and salt-free.

193 MORNING GLORY

Scientists have found that people who eat breakfast every day are a third less likely to be obese compared to those who skipped it, and are half as likely to have blood-sugar problems. Its also crucial to get the content of your breakfast bowl right since some cereals contain as much sugar as a chocolate bar and as much saturated fat as a portion of cake. The best option is to make your own porridge, using organically-grown oats sourced locally.

194 BECOME A MUESLI MIXER

Save money and gain peace of mind by mixing your own muesli. You'll also be able to ensure that the nuts, fruits, seeds and grains you choose are produced ethically and in a sustainable manner. Plus, by buying in bulk you'll be saving on packaging and reducing the carbon emissions that would have resulted from frequent purchases of pre-packed muesli.

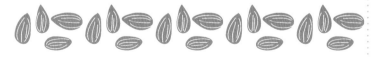

195 BARS ARE NOT THE ANSWER

More than half the UK population purchases a cereal bar every six weeks but replacing a nutritional breakfast with a cereal bar is unlikely to be helping you or the planet. Tests on cereal bars found them to be high in saturated fat and sugar. Then there's the packaging – each bar is individually wrapped – plus the energy used to process them.

196 A HEALTHY CUPPA

Researchers have indicated that tea could be just as good, if not better than water as it rehydrates the body and also provides valuable antioxidants, some minerals and is a natural source of fluoride which can help teeth. Drinking tea has been linked to a reduced risk of heart disease and some cancers, but don't drink it with a meal or just before or after as it can block the absorption of iron from food.

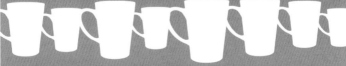

197 OPT FOR ORGANIC

When it comes to tea it's best to buy organic and fairtrade or teas that have met other high certification standards, such as those set by the Rainforest Alliance. Non-organic tea plantations are heavy users of pesticides and will often pay workers below a minimum wage. Plus, of the 132 million children estimated to be working in agriculture by the International Labour Organization, many are working on tea plantations.

198 LOOSEN UP

It's better to buy loose tea than tea in bags since less there is less packaging involved and ultimately fewer resources are used. There may also be a case for saying that loose-leaf teas are often better quality than those teas that make it into bags. But if you do buy bags, look for those produced with unbleached paper.

199 HEALTHY HERBALS

Herbal teas or infusions have been used to treat a huge variety of ailments for centuries. Made from the roots, flowers, bark, seeds, stems or leaves of herbs and spices, they contain no caffeine. But many herbal infusions may contain residues from agricultural chemicals while others might have been unsustainably harvested from the wild. Opt for organic with as little packaging as possible, or, better still, make your own by infusing the leaves or flowers in boiling water for 3 to 5 minutes.

200 FRUITY FACTS

Fruit teas or infusions aren't always packed full of the fruits that appear on their labels. For example, the Food Commission found that some cranberry, strawberry and raspberry tea bags contained only 0.2% strawberry. Ask the manufacturers where the flavour is actually coming from and don't be fooled into thinking you'll get the same benefits as you would from actually eating a piece of fresh fruit.

201 THE BEST CAFFEINE FIX

Coffee's contribution to carbon dioxide emissions is minimal because the plant captures and holds carbon in its woody stem and roots throughout its life. It's the chemicals used to grow it and the large amounts of water used to extract the beans from the pods that are the environmental bad guys.

202 COFFEE CAUTION

Like tea, coffee is another commodity that brings big profits to the brand owners but barely a living wage for many of the 25 million people in the tropics that depend on coffee farming. A good way to be sure that growers get a fair return is to buy products labelled 'fairtrade' – this not only guarantees a minimum price for suppliers, but also pays an extra premium for farmers to invest in community projects and encourages sustainable methods of farming.

203 GREEN ORIGINS?

Make sure your coffee supplier really knows where their beans have come from. The World Wildlife Fund recently found that some coffee brands contained coffee that was illegally grown inside one of the world's most important national parks for highly endangered tigers, elephants and rhinos. In its report, 'Gone in an Instant', WWF said that most of the companies buying the coffee were unaware of its illegal origins.

204 SEEK OUT THE SHADE

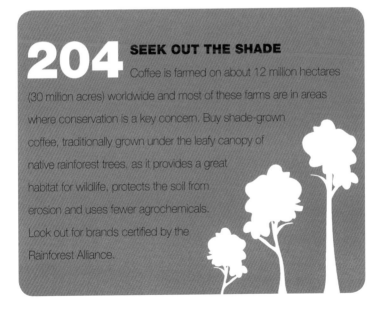

Coffee is farmed on about 12 million hectares (30 million acres) worldwide and most of these farms are in areas where conservation is a key concern. Buy shade-grown coffee, traditionally grown under the leafy canopy of native rainforest trees, as it provides a great habitat for wildlife, protects the soil from erosion and uses fewer agrochemicals. Look out for brands certified by the Rainforest Alliance.

205 BBQ WITH CAUTION

Don't be tempted by too many barbecues this summer. The smoke not only produces hydrocarbons but also tiny soot particles that pollute the air and can aggravate heart and lung problems. Also, meat cooked on a barbecue can form potentially cancer-causing compounds – the hotter the temperature and the longer the meat cooks, the more compounds produced.

206 GREEN BBQS

If you do indulge in a bit of barbecue action, then make sure you use locally produced charcoal from sustainable sources; avoid briquettes (the US Environmental Protection Agency says charcoal briquettes release 105 times more carbon monoxide per unit of energy than propane and a lot of toxic volatile organic compounds) and ditch the disposable – it's a massive waste of resources.

207 ENJOY IN MODERATION

There's no denying the terrible impact alcohol can have on people's health – it has been linked with an increased risk of mouth and throat cancers; it can also cause ulcers, liver disease, high blood pressure … the list goes on. Yet, recent Danish research found that people who led an active lifestyle and drank moderately (at least one drink per week) were less prone to heart disease.

208 DRINK A LOCAL TIPPLE

The export of beers and wines all over the world comes at a cost in terms of CO_2 emissions. Seek out your local breweries and vineyards. In England and Wales there are nearly 400 commercial vineyards (find them on www.english-wine.com), while in the US there are more than 1,300 independent, traditional 'craft' breweries (www.beertown.org).

209 AN ORGANIC ALE

Your regular beer could be made with hops that have been sprayed up to 14 times each year with an average of 15 pesticide products. Organic beer is made from organic malt and hops using farming methods that rule out this kind of chemical saturation. Look out also for 'carbon neutral beer' – Adnams brewery in the UK uses an Energy Recovery System that recycles 100% of the steam created during the brewing process and uses it to heat 90% of the following brew.

210 FINE WINE

A study by the European Pesticides Action Network (PAN) has found that wines on sale in the EU may contain residues of up to 10 different pesticides potentially harmful to human health. According to PAN, grapes receive a higher dose of synthetic pesticides than almost any other crop. To avoid guzzling pesticide residues in your wine, buy organic.

211 WHAT'S IN YOUR GLASS?

As well as possible pesticide residues, most wines contain additives which, unlike food, do not have to be listed on the label. These include fining agents, such as isinglass, which is made from fish bladders, clay or silica as well as sulphur, which is used as a preservative, ascorbic or tartaric acid, and sugar to increase the alcohol content. Certified organic wines add less sulphur dioxide to the wine – on average organic producers use just one quarter of the legal maximum for conventional wines.

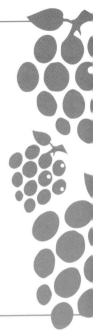

212 HAVE A CORKING TIME

Make sure your wine has a real cork, rather than a plastic one or screw top. You will be supporting the cork industry, one of the most environmentally friendly industries, which helps to maintain endangered wildlife such as the Iberian lynx, Spanish Imperial eagle and Barbary deer, while also cutting back on your plastic consumption.

213 A LIGHTER DRINK

Some retailers have started using lighter glass bottles for wines, which need less energy to transport, while other wines are packaged in cartons made from renewable materials, which are also a lighter load. Given that in most countries a large proportion of the wine is imported, choosing the lightest possible packaging will help reduce your carbon footprint. Look out too for imported wines that are bottled closer to home so cutting needless transport emissions.

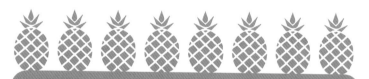

214 RAISE YOUR SPIRITS

Even hardened liquor drinkers can be eco-friendly by opting for organic and ethically sourced spirits. In the case of rum, it is sugar that is the principle ingredient and which should come from a sustainable source, while with vodka the grain that is used could have been drenched in pesticides. Check the brand's website to see if they state the source of their key ingredient.

215 WILD GIN

In many areas wild sloes – the fruit of the blackthorn (*Prunus spinosa*) – are readily available and can be used to flavour gin. Just prick the skins with a needle, add 250 g (½ lb) sugar for each 500 g (1 lb) sloes, fill a bottle halfway with the sloes and top up with gin. Shake, store and turn occasionally and the gin should be ready in a couple of months. Strain first, then drink as an after-dinner liqueur or mix with white wine or champagne.

216 SOYA SAGA

Soya, in its various forms, can be found in more than 60% of processed food such as breakfast cereals, biscuits, cakes, gravies, pastries and sauces. But growing demand has led to the destruction of large swathes of precious South American habitat and is one of the main threats to the Amazon rainforest. So cut out processed food and cut back on cheap meat too – the demand for soya in animal feed is also driving deforestation.

217 SOYA RISK

Being high in omega-6 fatty acids, soya is thought to be one of the reasons why our balance of omega-3 to omega-6 essential fatty acids is so out of kilter, plus it has a high content of phytoestrogens, which can mimic or block the action of the human hormone oestrogen. Those with a thyroid problem and women with oestrogen-dependent breast cancer are particularly at risk from a diet high in soya.

218 VEGGIES BEWARE

While it is a great idea to give beefburgers a miss, replacing them with veggie burgers may not be the best alternative. Many of these are made with soya-based Textured Vegetable Protein, which needs a lot of energy to produce and is far from a traditional natural product. Choose organic varieties made with rice, beans and/or vegetables.

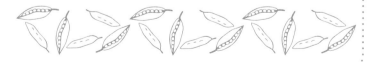

219

TRADITIONAL PRACTICES

When buying soya products, such as soya sauce or miso, select those that have been made according to traditional methods from Japan and China, whereby the soya has been fermented for months. This process reduces the levels of the phytoestogens by two- to threefold and saves on fossil fuels used in modern factory processing. Plus, Japanese or Chinese strains of soya have lower levels of isoflavones. Beware non-brewed soya sauce, which is made in just two days and will have salt, caramel and chemical preservatives and flavourings added to provide colour and taste.

220

SAVE ON SUPPLEMENTS

A well-balanced diet, one that is high in fruit and vegetables, should be enough to keep most of us healthy. Occasionally, there may be an advantage to taking a supplement – folic acid when pregnant, for example, but otherwise save on the natural resources and energy needed to produce, package and distribute them.

221 FISH-OIL FEARS

Fish oils are not only sold as supplements, but are also added to animal and farmed fish feed. But some can contain potentially pollutants such as dioxins and polychlorinated biphenyls (PCBs) and they can also come from unsustainable fishery operations. Check the purity and sustainability of any fish oils you buy and consider safer options such as flaxseed oil or algae-derived sources of omega-3s.

222 RADIATION CONCERNS

A few years ago a UK government survey found that nearly half the food supplements sampled were completely irradiated (see tip 249) or contained an irradiated ingredient but were not labelled as such. Several studies link irradiation with a reduction in nutritional value, but it's also a reminder that supplements are essentially processed products.

223 BUY NATURAL SUPPLEMENTS

If you do need to take a food supplement, beware those made with synthetic nutrients that are manufactured using chemicals. In the US, the Organic Consumers Association says that 90% or more of the vitamins and supplements now on the market labelled as 'natural' or 'food-based' are actually spiked with synthetic chemicals. It is developing a new set of Naturally Occurring Standards (NOS), which will lead to the certification of genuinely natural products – see www.organicconsumers.org/nutricon.cfm.

224 SUSTAINABLE SOURCING

The demand for herbal remedies in North America and Europe has been growing by about 10% a year for the last decade but it is now threatening to wipe out 10,000 of the world's 50,000 medicinal plant species, according to Plantlife International. Ask the retailer where the raw material for your herbal remedy comes from and how it's harvested.

225 CHOCOLATE HEAVEN

Research has shown that eating small amounts of chocolate with a high cocoa content could bring nutritional benefits such as lower blood pressure and a reduced risk of death from cardiovascular disease because the chocolate is rich in antioxidants (flavonoids) and trace minerals. However, chocolate is also high in sugar and saturated fat, so consume high-cocoa-content chocolate in moderation.

226 SAVE THE TROPICS

Over 18 million acres (7.5 million hectares) of tropical land is used to grow cocoa so the way it is produced effects a big chunk of habitat. Like coffee, it is best for biodiversity to buy cocoa that has been grown under the shade of native canopy trees in a landscape similar to natural forest. It is also good to buy organic and fairtrade chocolate as cocoa crops may be heavily sprayed with agrochemicals, while plantation workers can be working in conditions akin to slave labour.

227 SWEET AS HONEY

For thousands of years, honey has been used as a natural remedy for ailments – from sore throats to burns and cuts – because of its antiseptic properties. And this is one product that most of us can source locally. Supporting local, small-scale beekeepers will cut your food miles and ensure bees continue to play their vital role in pollinating crops in the countryside near you.

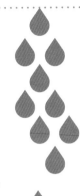

228 EXOTIC IMPORTS

If you can't source locally produced honey, then opt for fairtrade and/or organic honey from overseas rather than mainstream commercial products. Commercial beekeepers may use synthetic pesticides and antibiotics to combat pests, while organic bees can't be treated with antibiotics as they must be able to forage in organically cultivated areas or areas of natural vegetation free from pesticides.

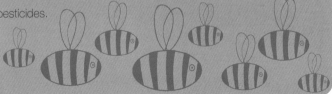

229 GO FOR JARS

Ignore the ads enticing you to pick 'easy squeeze' plastic bottles for your condiments and spreads. It is better to go for glass jars, especially those with a high recycled content (ask the manufacturer or retailer). In most countries, they can be recycled more easily than plastic and you can re-use them.

230 BEE FRIENDLY

Honeybees are big business – in the UK, bees contribute £165 million a year to the economy through their pollination of fruit trees, field beans and other crops, while in the US bee pollination services are worth an estimated $15 billion. But they are currently disappearing – almost two million colonies of honeybees have disappeared in the US. Pesticides are likely to be part of the problem, so help by supporting organic agriculture (see www.aworldwithoutbees.com).

231 GET SAUCY

There's been a shift away from glass bottles to plastic bottles in the world of sauces and condiments. Packaging already represents the largest single sector of plastics used and, even if your local authority will recycle plastic, the recycling process is more complex and energy intensive than it is for glass. Whether it's ketchup or mayonnaise, avoid adding to the plastic mountain and stick to glass bottles. Even better – make your own condiments.

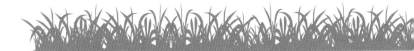

232 GROW YOUR OWN JUICE

Wheatgrass is packed with vitamins, minerals, enzymes and chlorophyll and makes a healthy juice. Try growing your own wheatgrass to prepare your own juice – you can purchase kits with organic seeds and compost online to make it even easier.

233 GET JUICING

Give your body a treat and invest in a juicer. It's a great way of getting your five-a-day of fresh fruit and vegetables and ensures you have a concentrated source of minerals, vitamins and enzymes. In fact, liquidizing or juicing can increase the availability of some substances, such as carotenoids from carrots. Make sure you include a mix of ingredients such as beetroot, spinach and carrots, or apple, celery and lemon; remember to put the waste pulp and skin on your compost heap, too.

234 ARE YOU GETTING FRESH?

Most shop-bought juices have been pasteurized – a process which kills bacteria and germs but which many believe can destroy vitamins, minerals and enzymes. Plus fruit sugars in the whole fruit are less damaging to teeth than those released during processing. A manual juice press or simple juice squeezer needs no electricity and you will get a fresh, vitamin-packed drink.

235 THE TRUE COST OF OJ

Chances are your orange juice will have travelled miles before it ends up in your fridge – 80% of orange juice consumed in Europe comes from Brazil, and Brazil and Florida now grow between them nearly half the world's oranges, 95% of which are juiced. As well as all those transport emissions, a study has found that for every glass of Brazilian orange juice drunk, 22 glasses of processing water and 1,000 glasses of irrigation water are required. Choose juices made from local fruits instead.

236 SAY NO TO SODA

Fizzy drinks or sodas account for over 28% of all drinks consumed in the US and it is thought that the average American teenage boy drinks 3.5 cans of soda each day, while one in ten drinks 7 cans a day. But soda is empty of nutritional value and high in sugar and potentially harmful chemicals, such as the preservative sodium benzoate. Plus, even if you recycle the can, the energy and resources gobbled up by the soda industry is still incredibly wasteful. Do yourself a favour and have a glass of water instead.

237

CHECK THE BACTERIA

Those little plastic bottles of probiotic health drinks are popular, but they may not always be accepted for recycling, and there are concerns about some less well-known brands. Studies have found that one in two probiotic health drinks tested do not have the healthy bacteria claimed on the label, while others contain a type of bacteria that's unlikely to survive in the gut. Look for those containing *lactobacilli* or *bifidobacterium*, and a minimum of 10 million bacteria per bottle.

238

NUTS ABOUT NUTS

Research has shown that eating nuts five or more times a week can reduce the risk of heart attack by 60% and there are many other health benefits. They may be high in fat, but people who regularly eat nuts are also more likely to be lean than those who don't. But check the nuts you buy are organic, as pesticides are commonly used in production.

239 SUNNY SIDE OF SEEDS

Whether it's from your sunflowers or pumpkins, remember you can harvest the seeds to make a nutritious snack. In the case of the sunflower, once it has finished flowering tie a paper bag over the flower to catch the seeds as they dry. Try roasting the dry seeds or, if you have enough of them, remove the hulls and crush them to make a tasty nut butter.

240 GROW YOUR OWN SPICES

Spices usually come from tropical countries, but it is perfectly possible to grow some of your own and cut down on your food miles. Coriander seed, chilli peppers and curry leaf – *murraya koenigii* – will all grow in temperate climates if you can find a suitably sunny spot and keep the plants frost-free.

241 SPICE UP YOUR LIFE

Spices not only add flavour, they can also provide valuable health benefits. Turmeric, for example, has antioxidant, anticancer and anti-inflammatory properties, while cinnamon is thought to protect against type II diabetes and heart disease. Buy whole dried spices and grind them yourself in an energy-saving pestle and mortar to get the best flavour.

242 BEST SPICES

Seek out organic and fairtrade spices. Not only will you avoid pesticide residues and be certain the growers are receiving a fair price for their labour, but you will also be sure that the spices have not been irradiated (see tips 249 and 250). Irradiation of spices on a commercial scale is practised in over 20 countries and in 2000, 80,000 metric tonnes of spice were processed worldwide using irradiation, yet there have been no studies on the long-term effects of eating irradiated food.

243 PROTEIN FROM PULSES

Substituting pulses (legumes) for meat could bring down the climate cost of our diets (see tips 82 and 84). Choose from a range of beans, peas and lentils and add them to stews, casseroles, soups and sauces or use them in salads. They are high in fibre, which may help lower blood cholesterol, and a good source of iron (although try to drink orange juice or eat foods high in vitamin C with them in order to help absorb the iron).

244 BEANS AT HOME

Grow and dry your own pulses and enjoy an incredible array of beans in all sizes and colours. First, source varieties marked as suitable for drying, often from heritage seed suppliers such as www.heritageharvestseed.com. Once the plants have grown, just leave the pods on the plant – when they're brown, dry and rattling, the beans can be removed from the pods and packed in airtight jars.

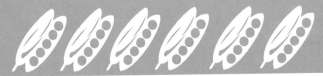

245
ARTISAN ICE CREAM

Some non-dairy ice creams contain palm oil – listed as 'vegetable fat', while other ingredients might include chemical colourings, emulsifiers, stabilizers and partially hydrogenated fats, as well as a lot of air to add bulk (up to 120% air in cheap ice cream). Look for artisan dairy ice creams made using natural, organic and authentic eggs, milk and cream.

246
YUMMY YOGURT

Yogurt is rich in protein, B vitamins and calcium but make sure you pick an organic brand in order to avoid artificial additives, flavourings, sweeteners, and so on. You can also benefit from the higher omega-3 fatty acids and antioxidants commonly found in organic milk (see tip 110). Choose yogurts that are low in sugar.

247 GET READY FOR CLONES

Regulatory authorities in the US and Europe have decided that meat and milk from cloned cattle is safe, and a ban on the sale of cloned food in the US has been lifted. Already claims are being made for cloning, such as the possibility of cloning a cow that produces lower-fat milk, but others argue that there isn't enough evidence to be certain about the long-term health effects and that cloning reduces biodiversity.

248 SAY NO TO NANO

The food industry is busy researching the use of nanotechnology in ingredients, additives and packaging. There are the usual promises of environmental and health benefits – products may be able to adjust their nutrient content to meet each consumer's health needs, for example. But many scientific institutions are worried about the lack of research into the safety. For more information see www.nanotechproject.org and http://nano.foe.org.au.

249 SPREADING IRRADIATION

Food irradiation – where food is exposed to high doses of ionizing radiation that kills insects, moulds and bacterium – is being promoted, especially in the US, as the answer to food poisoning and for extending food shelf life. But some believe that it can result in loss of nutrients and mask poor hygiene practices in food production by sterilizing contamination. Look at the label: US federal rules require irradiated foods to be labelled as such.

250 MORE ON IRRADIATION

On the environmental side, there are risks of pollution from radioactive irradiation plants and the fact that irradiation allows food to be transported over greater distances. Currently, only herbs, spices and vegetable seasonings are irradiated in Europe but in the US the list of foods is longer and includes wheat, potatoes, fruit and vegetables, herbs and spices, pork, poultry and beef. The sure way to avoid it is to buy organic, which bans irradiation. See www.organicconsumers.org/irradlink.cfm.